The Louisiana State Bird Beauty Pageant

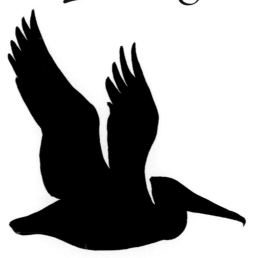

Written by Todd-Michael St. Pierre
Illustrated by Lori Walsh

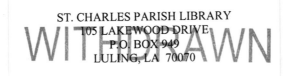

Second Printing

Published by:

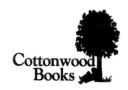

**Cottonwood
Books**

3054 Perkins Rd.
Baton Rouge, LA 70808
225-343-1266

In association with WordBlossoms.com

Library of Congress Catalog Card Number: 00-191007
International Standard Book Number: 0-9675170-0-1

Printed by:
Starr★Toof Printing

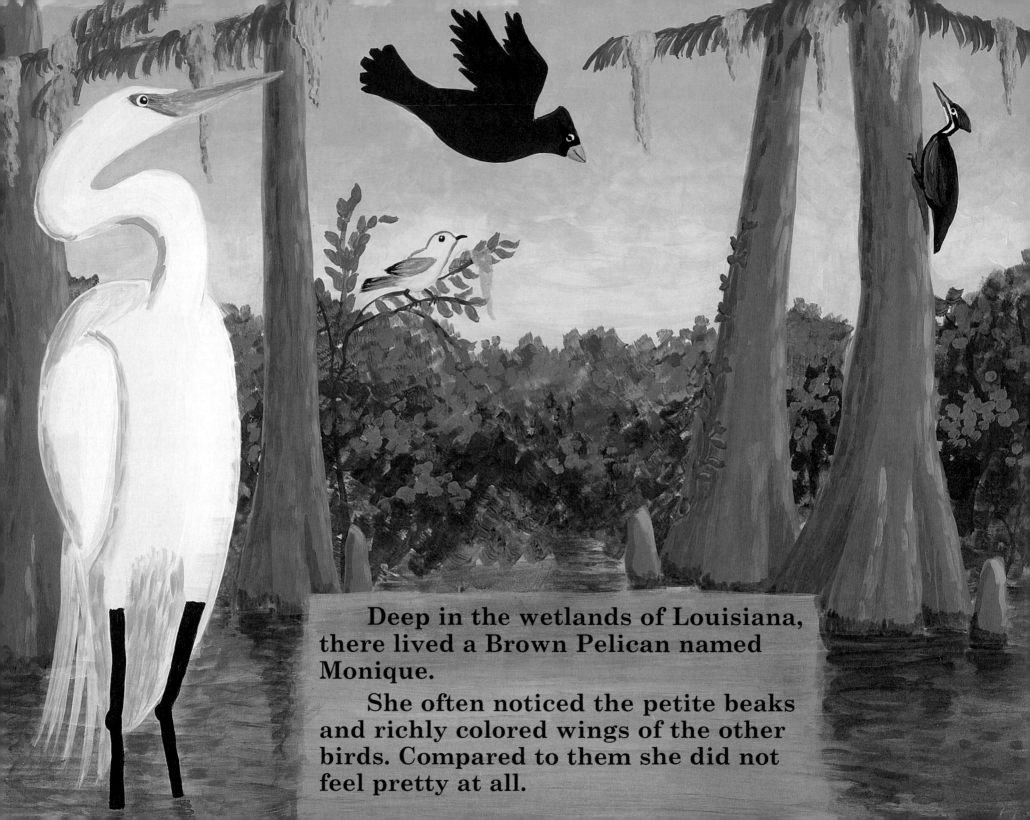

Deep in the wetlands of Louisiana, there lived a Brown Pelican named Monique.

She often noticed the petite beaks and richly colored wings of the other birds. Compared to them she did not feel pretty at all.

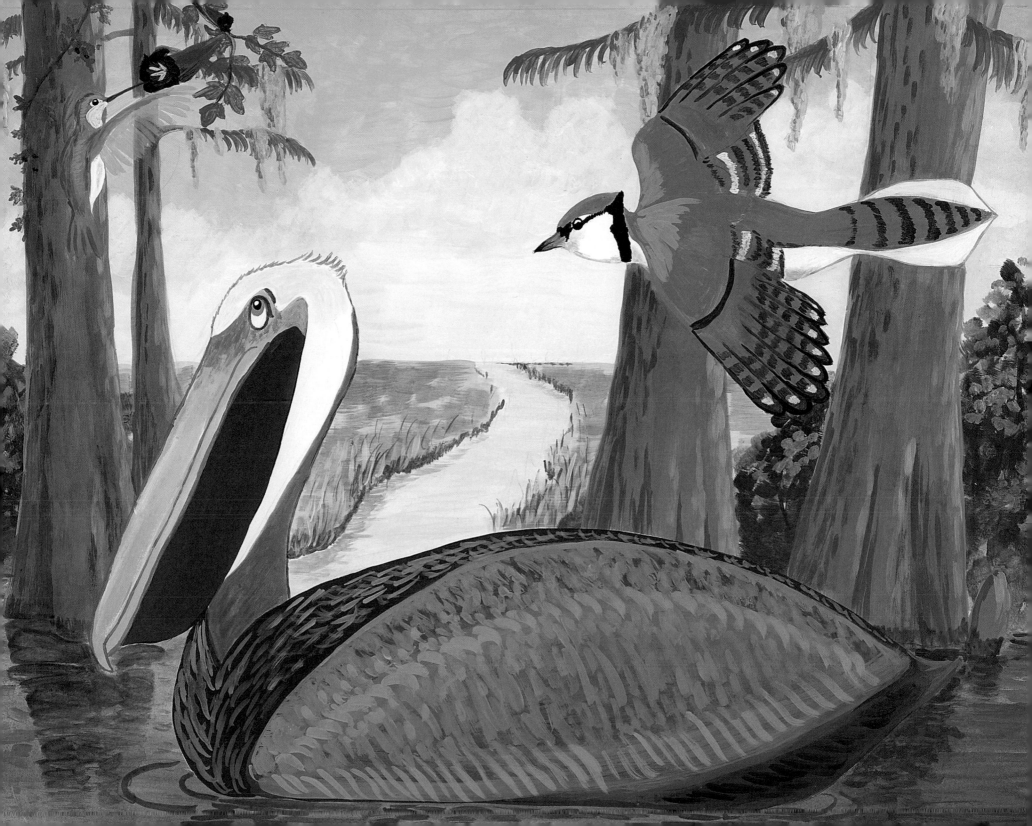

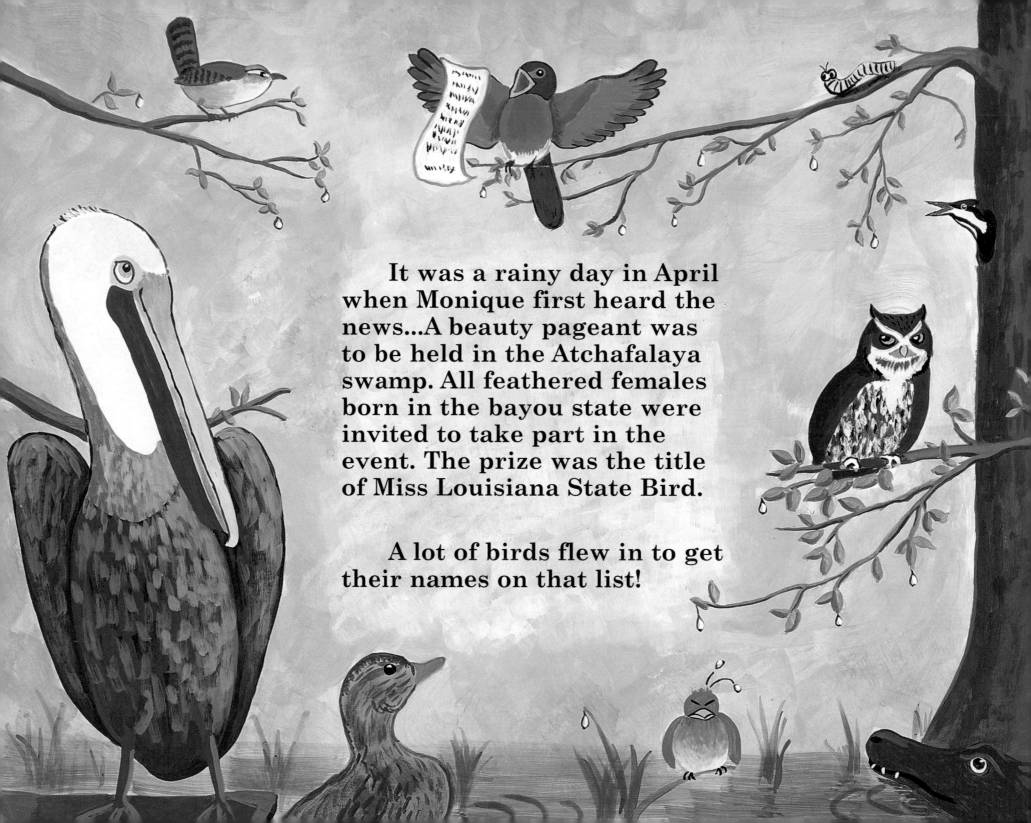

It was a rainy day in April when Monique first heard the news...A beauty pageant was to be held in the Atchafalaya swamp. All feathered females born in the bayou state were invited to take part in the event. The prize was the title of Miss Louisiana State Bird.

A lot of birds flew in to get their names on that list!

Calling All Sixty-Four Parishes

The Louisiana State Bird Beauty Pageant.
Oh, it's almost here.
It's a bird bonanza, extravaganza,
And the day is getting near.
Seeking contestants in all shapes and sizes,
And we don't have lots of time.
Your face on the flag and fabulous prizes.
What a chance to shine!
It's a rare and splendid opportunity,
Coming soon to our community.
That day is getting near.
The Louisiana State Bird Beauty Pageant.
Oh, it's almost here.

P.S. No Mosquitoes, Please!

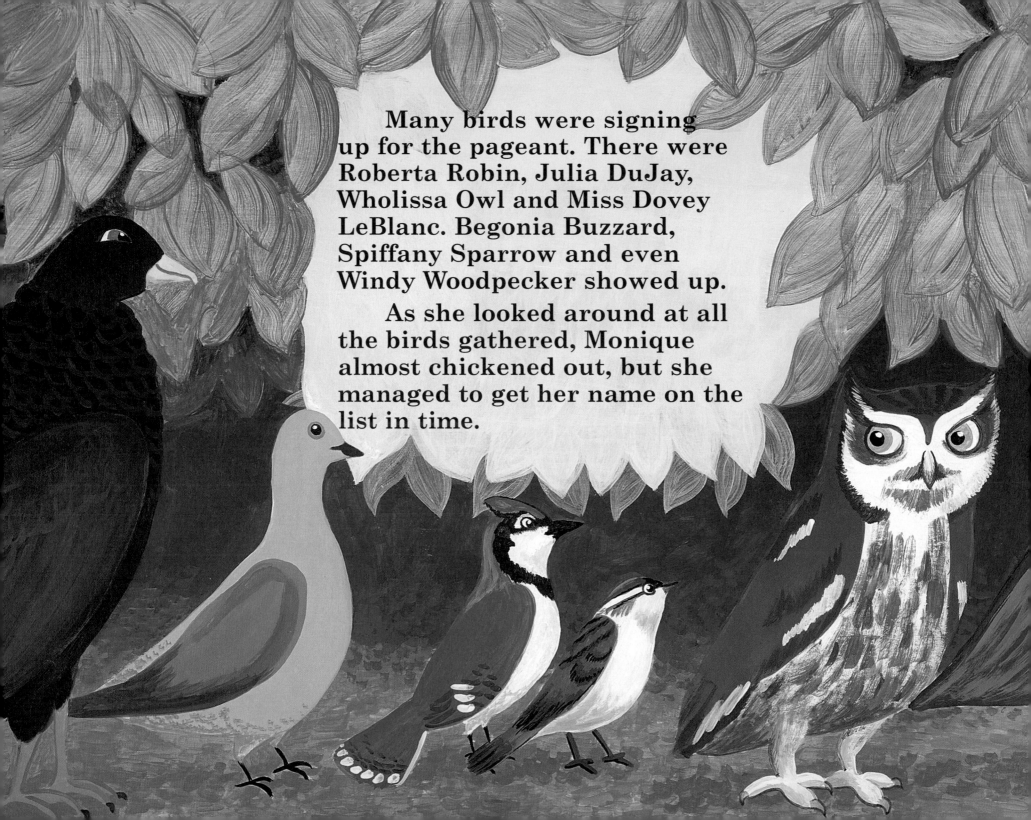

Many birds were signing up for the pageant. There were Roberta Robin, Julia DuJay, Wholissa Owl and Miss Dovey LeBlanc. Begonia Buzzard, Spiffany Sparrow and even Windy Woodpecker showed up.

As she looked around at all the birds gathered, Monique almost chickened out, but she managed to get her name on the list in time.

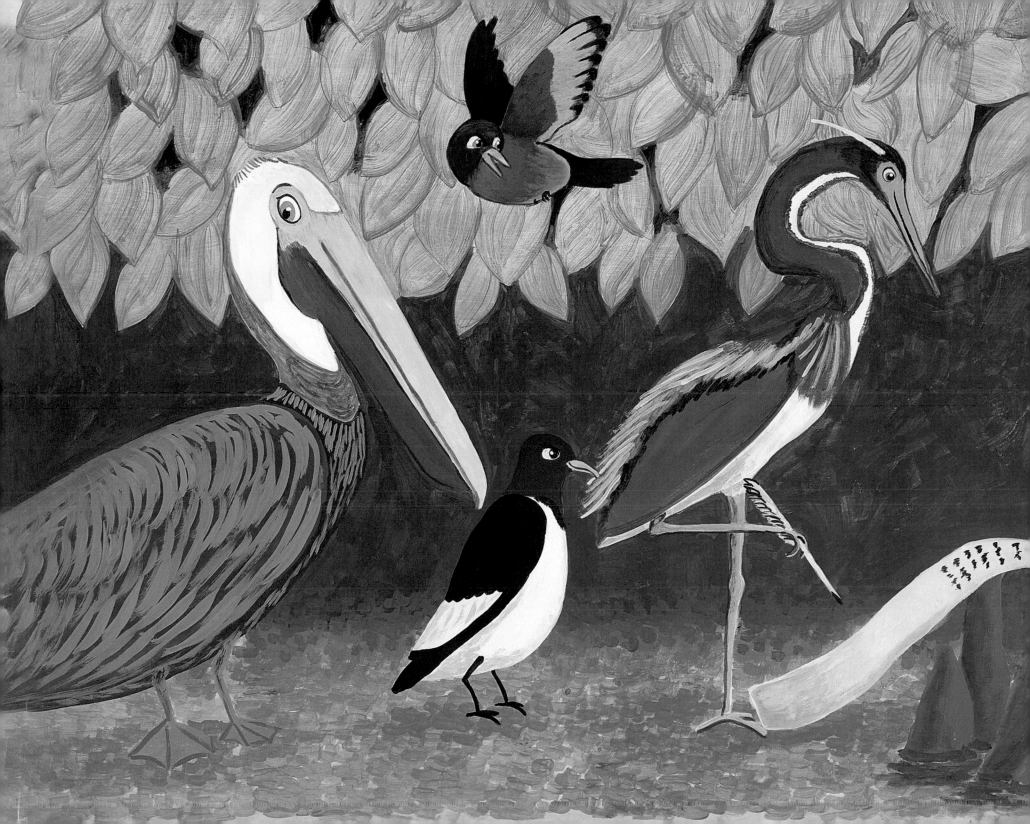

The following Saturday Monique went to the annual "For The Birds" crawfish boil. And that is when the teasing and mean jokes began.

"You're not really going to be a contestant are you?" asked Carlotta Cardinal.

"There's a reason they call it a BEAUTY pageant," smirked Renée Wren.

"Your bill's too big and you wobble when you walk," said Yvette Egret.

Just then Magnolia Mockingbird shouted, "Hey girls, listen to this one! 'The pellycan, the pellycan, her bill holds more than her belly can'"

The birds chirped loudly, as they repeated the silly rhyme. "The pellycan, the pellycan, her bill holds more than her belly can!"

They laughed until Monique began to cry and she finally fled for home.

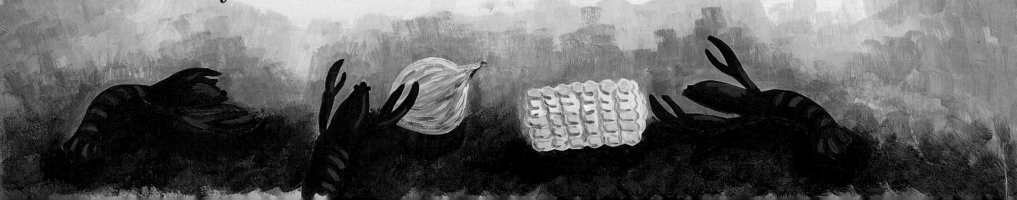

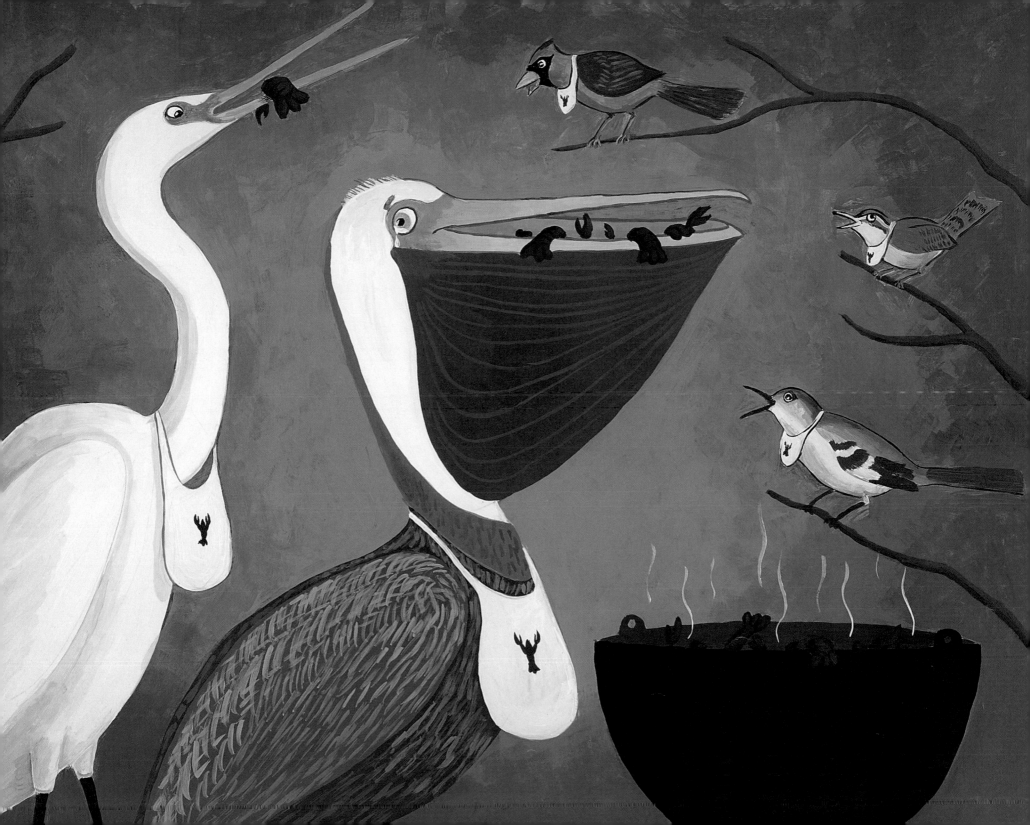

The next morning Monique decided to pay a visit to her friend Marie LaCrow. Marie was known throughout Cajun Country for her magic. Monique hoped that Marie could make her beautiful before the pageant.

"She must have a spell or a potion that will do the trick," thought Monique, as she knocked on the door of Marie's cypress shack.

When Marie saw Monique she knew that something was troubling her.

"You don't seem like yourself today. What is wrong?" questioned Marie.

It's the State Bird Beauty Pageant," answered Monique, as she began to cry again. "The others tease me because I'm plain and awkward."

"Nonsense," replied Marie. "I have always thought you were beautiful!"

With these words she handed Monique a necklace and she added, "This is a gris-gris, a charm my mother gave me long ago. Now I will pass it on to you. It will bring you luck; however, you must remember that true beauty comes from within. Believe me...THE MAGIC IS INSIDE OF YOU."

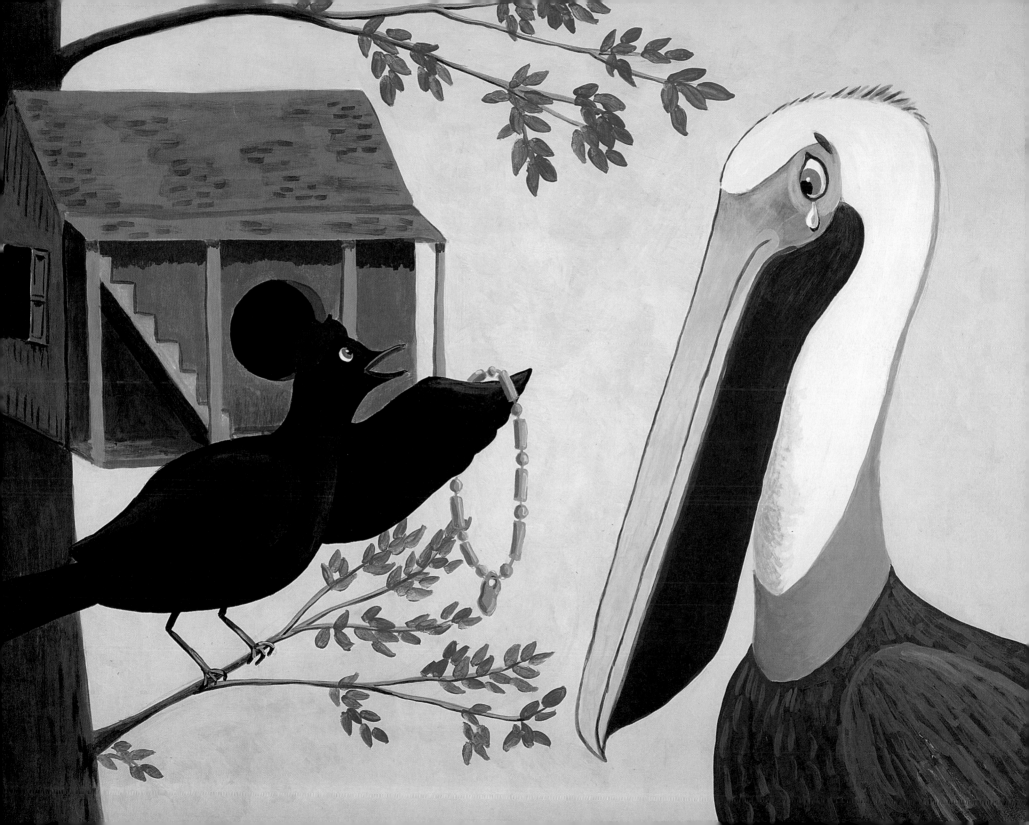

Then Marie sang these words to her...

"Be your own best friend, Monique.
They chirp and they chatter but that doesn't matter.
I think you are FANTASTIQUE!
If they tease then of course, please consider the source
And the nonsense they all speak.
There's a voice deep inside you, trust it to guide you...
I'm sure you'll see in the end,
This dream that you seek is a dream so unique.
Monique, be your own best friend!"

"I will try," promised Monique, as she put the charm around her neck. "Marie, you always know how to cheer me up," she said.

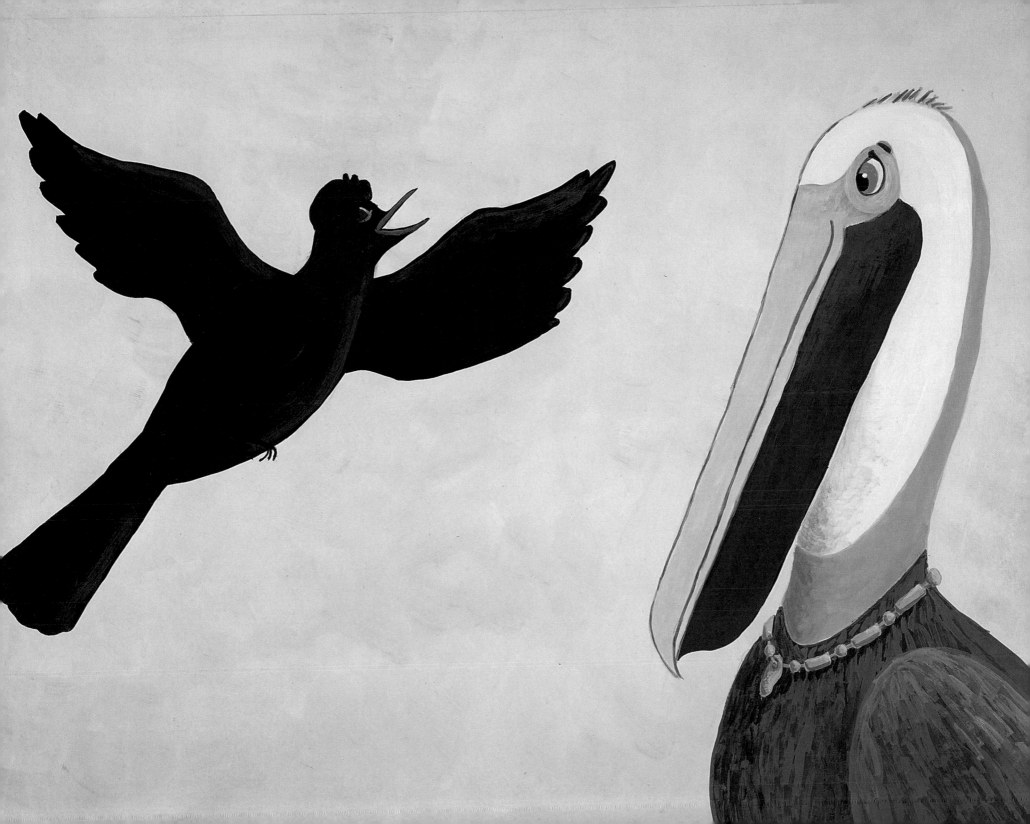

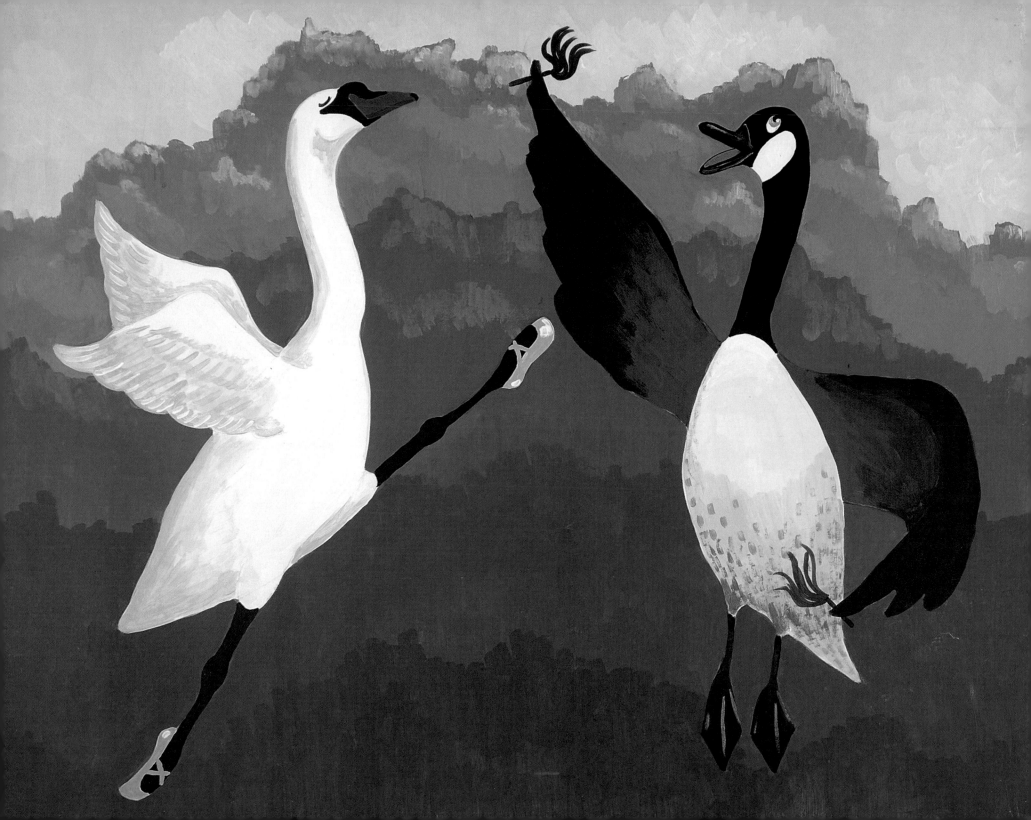

A month went by and soon the big day was one week away. Most of the contestants were busy rehearsing.

Gladiola Goose was showing off her cheerleading skills (tongue in beak). Helena Hummingbird went around giving samples of her acceptance speech to any creature who could stay awake long enough to hear the whole thing. Mignon La Swan declared that she could not lose with her Swan Lake ballet routine.

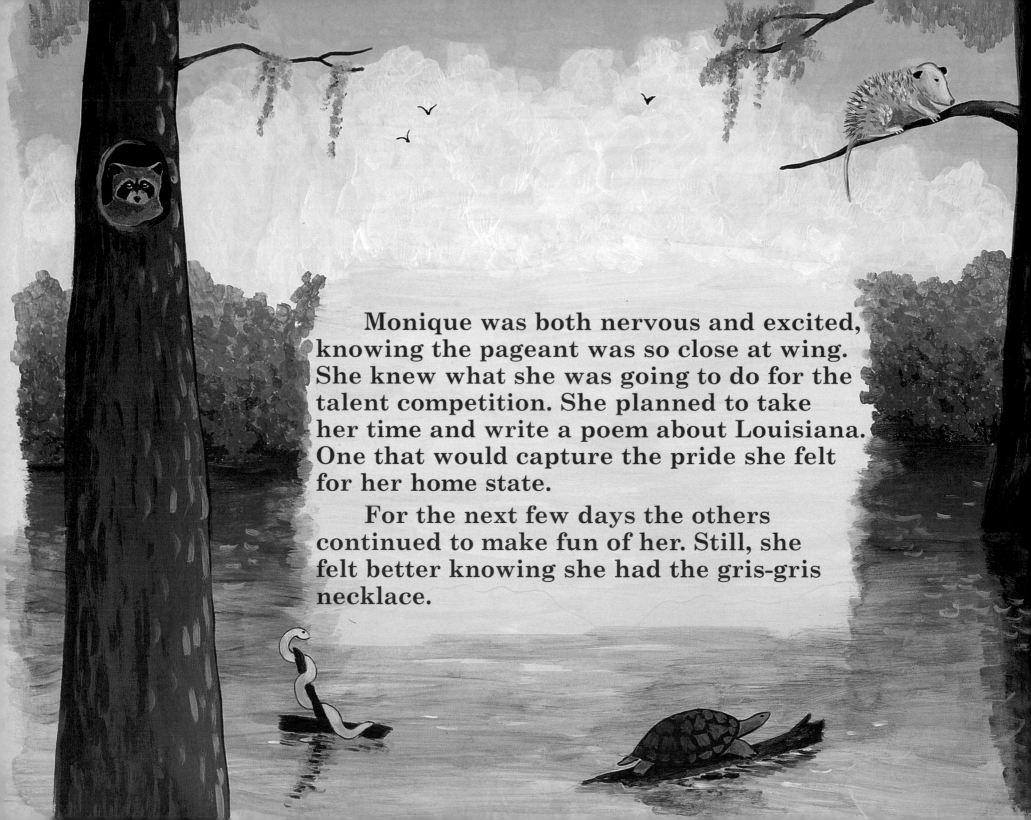

Monique was both nervous and excited, knowing the pageant was so close at wing. She knew what she was going to do for the talent competition. She planned to take her time and write a poem about Louisiana. One that would capture the pride she felt for her home state.

For the next few days the others continued to make fun of her. Still, she felt better knowing she had the gris-gris necklace.

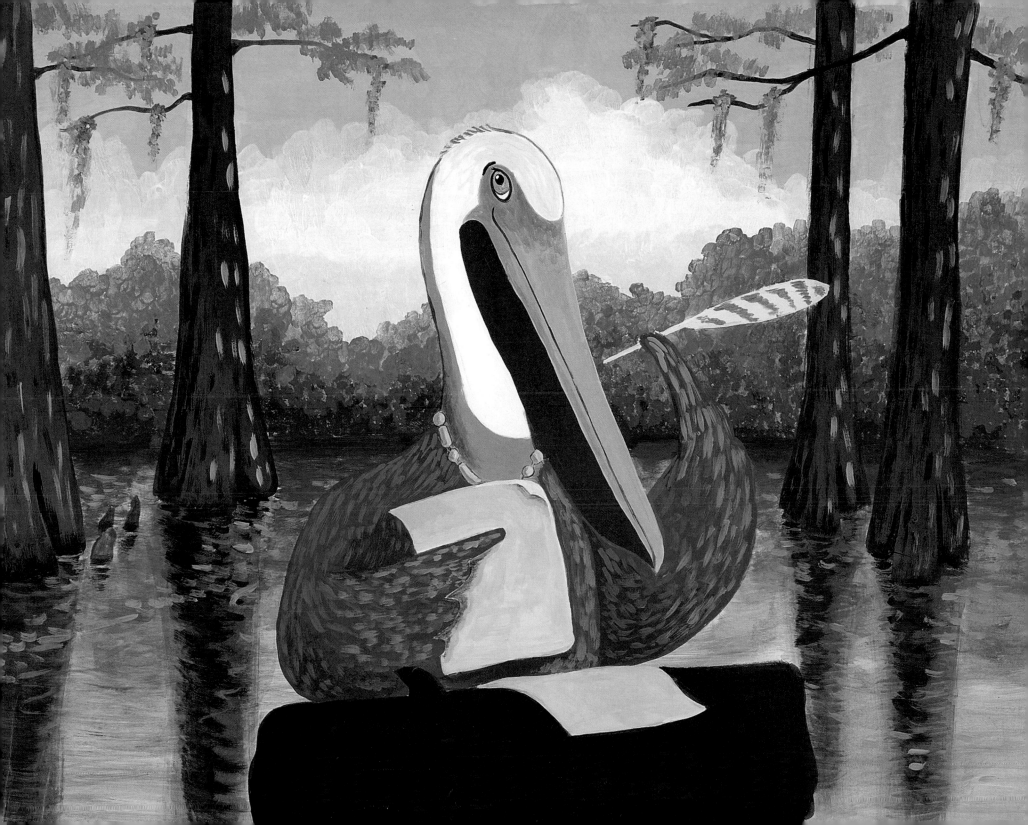

At last the day of the pageant had arrived. Monique had never seen so many birds in one place. Everybirdy was there to see who would be crowned Miss Louisiana State Bird.

When the others saw her they began to snicker and bicker. Julia DuJay started it.

"Monique, you might as well wobble on home. I intend to win this pageant! I paid a fortune for this pearl necklace," she bragged.

"Speaking of necklaces," said Dovey LeBlanc, "have y'all seen the one Monique is wearing? It's an outdated piece of junk," she laughed.

Begonia Buzzard joined in, "Monique as State Bird, now that's comedy!"

"It's not exactly an Audubon painting, that's for sure," chided Roberta Robin.

Then Wholissa Owl said, "Who does she think she is? Who would want a plain brown pelican to represent our state? Who?"

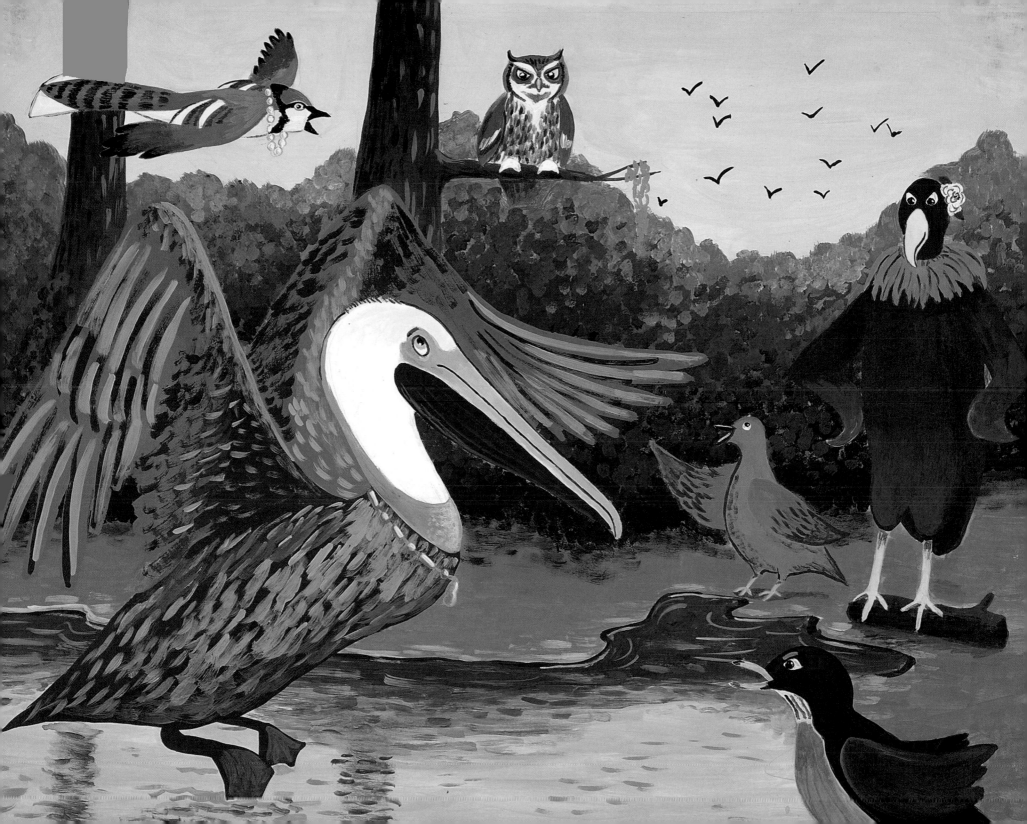

Marie LaCrow had just arrived and she had overheard their unkind words.

"What in the world are you girls doing?" asked Marie. "Have you no feelings?"

"We were just practicing," said Julia DuJay in a shaky, dishonest voice.

"That's not true," said Marie. " I heard what was said and you should all be ashamed."

Soon they scattered, leaving Monique and Marie to themselves.

"How can I go through with this?" asked Monique. "One minute I am sure of myself, then the next I'm scared."

"Don't you see?" asked Marie. "They behave that way because they are jealous."

"Jealous?" sobbed Monique, "Of me? I am nothing to be jealous of."

"Jealous of your inner beauty," Marie tried to explain. "All they have are fancy feathers and pretend smiles. But you have personality, talent, and intelligence. That frightens them! You are always helping others, like the time you flew Spiffany Sparrow to the hospital in Lafayette because she had broken a wing. I can still see you carrying the poor thing in your bill. And I'll never forget how you brought me gumbo when I was sick with the flu last year. Monique, you are the most unselfish and caring bird I know of. I see that as beautiful, and I have no doubt the judges will too!"

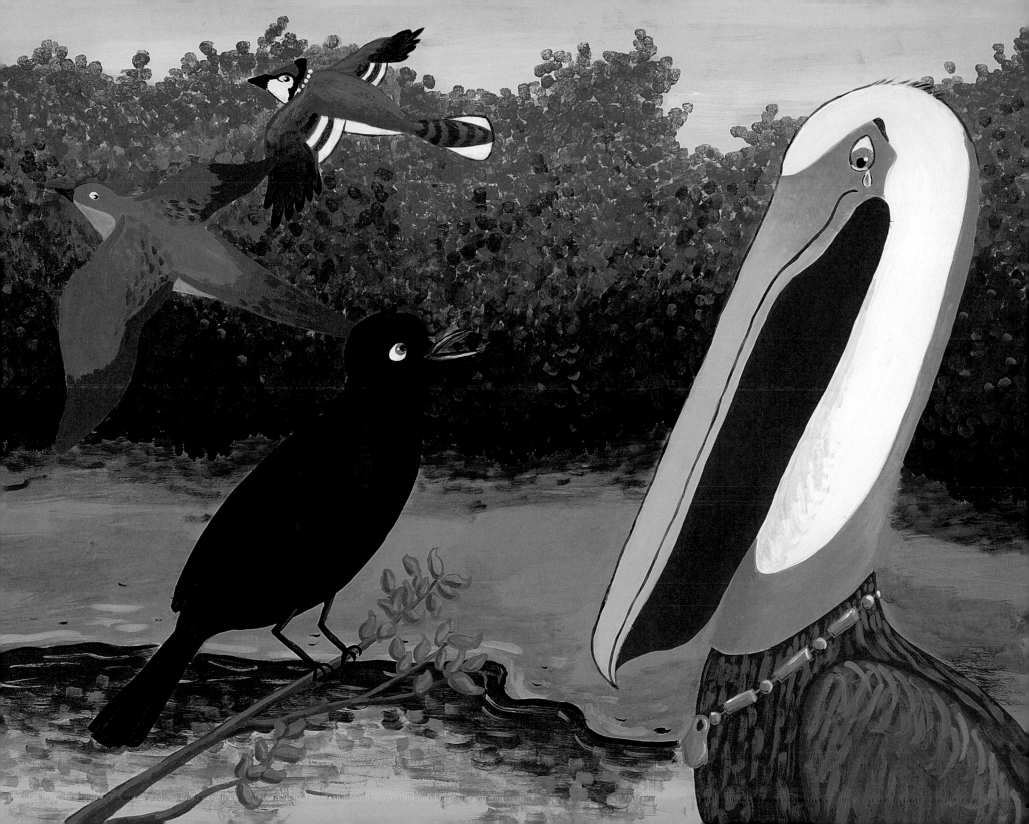

Marie continued. "So are you going to just stand there or are you going to get out there and shine? Like I said before...
THE MAGIC IS INSIDE OF YOU!"

Monique listened carefully. She knew that Marie was right. She had waited so long and had worked so hard on her poem, there was no turning back!

So she thanked Marie for her words of wisdom and for reminding her of how much the pageant meant to her.

Suddenly a voice from the stage announced that it was time for the talent competition. Pandora Pigeon of the French Quarter played the accordion. Her version of "*Jambalaya*" wasn't bad. Elaine Crane of White Castle did a rap version of "*You Are My Sunshine.*" It was interesting, to say the least! And those Blackbird twins, Zinnia and Gardenia, did a dramatic reading of Longfellow's "*Evangeline.*"

The pageant was only three hours long, but to Monique it seemed like forever. She was surprised at her own courage when it came time to read her poem...

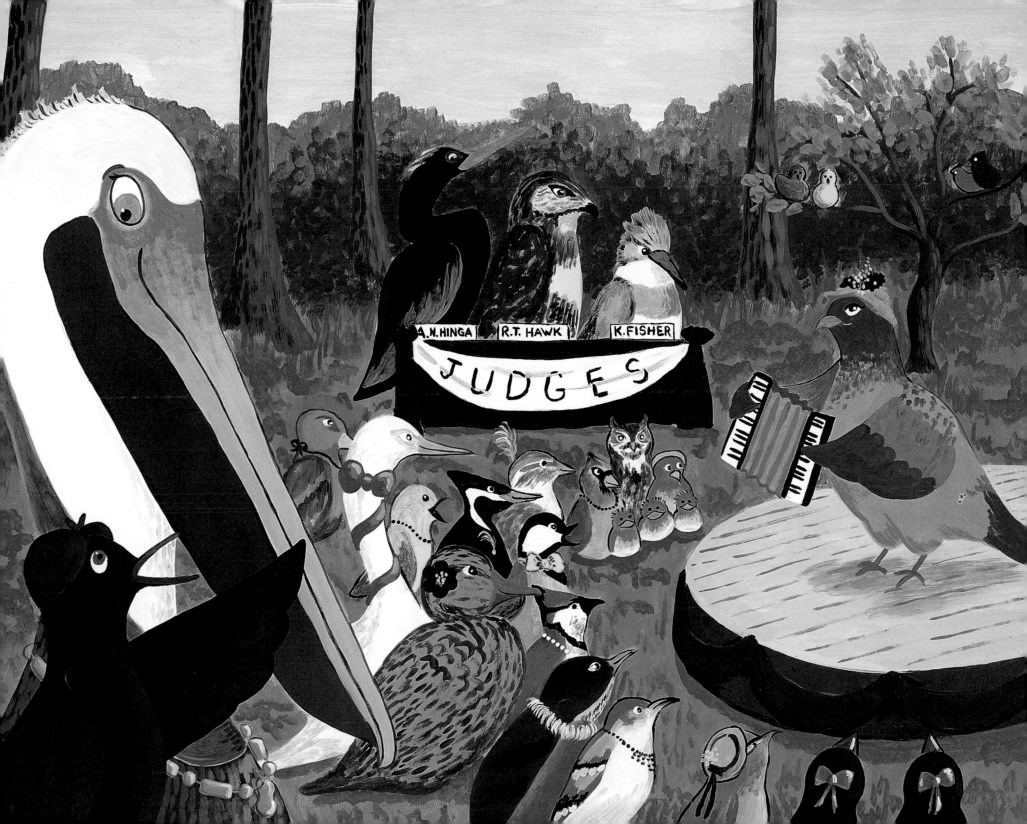

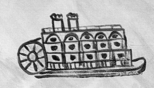
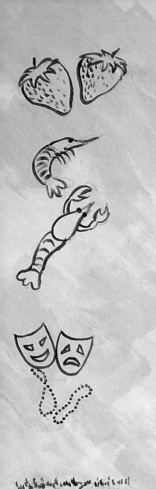

PRIDE

She is a lady. Her treasures I've seen.
Steamboats and *bonfires* and *Creole cuisine*,
Strawberries and seafood, sugarcane and rice,
Mardi Gras, cotton and hot *Cajun* spice,
Marshlands and campgrounds, *bayous* and beaches,
Melons, pecans and don't forget peaches.
She's the Belle of the Ball, what else can I say?
She's magic and music and *café au lait*.
Down by the levee near a plantation gate,
Where *pirogues* drift and festivals wait.
She's Spanish-moss mornings, a place I know well,
A walk by the river, a distant church bell.
She's *Zydeco*, Gospel, she's Blues and she's Jazz.
Just something about her no other state has.
It goes without saying, it's a feeling inside,
Louisiana my homeland, Louisiana my pride.

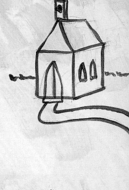
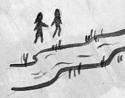
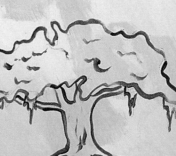
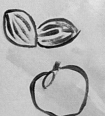
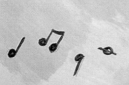

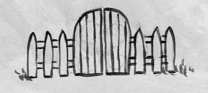
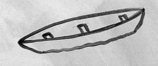

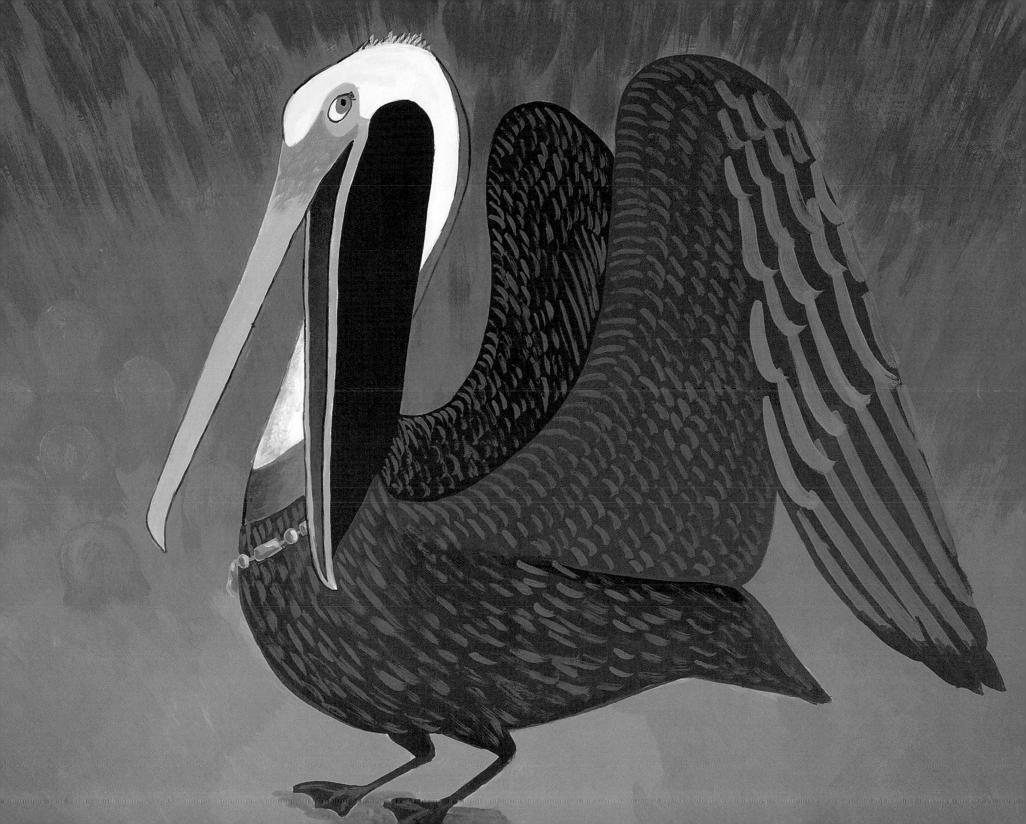

The audience loved it, and their applause was as loud as thunder. Marie gave her a hug as she left the stage and said, "I knew you could do it!"

After the final contestant finished the announcer asked... "Ladies and Gentlebirds, who do you think will be our State Bird?"

Monique took a deep breath.

The announcer continued, "We have some lovely and talented ladies with us here today. Yet, we can only have one winner. This is the moment we have all waited for. Judges, the envelope please."

There was complete silence as he opened it.

Then he spoke...

"Let's put our wings together for our official state bird, Miss Monique Pelican!"

"It worked," shouted Monique. "The gris-gris necklace, it really was magical, oh, Marie, how can I thank you?"

"No, no child," insisted Marie. "It was not the necklace! In your soul you have more power than any old hocus-pocus!"

The other birds were upset, some pouted and stomped, others cried and screamed. But in their hearts they knew that Monique Pelican was the best choice, for even though they had treated her so badly, Monique forgave them all.

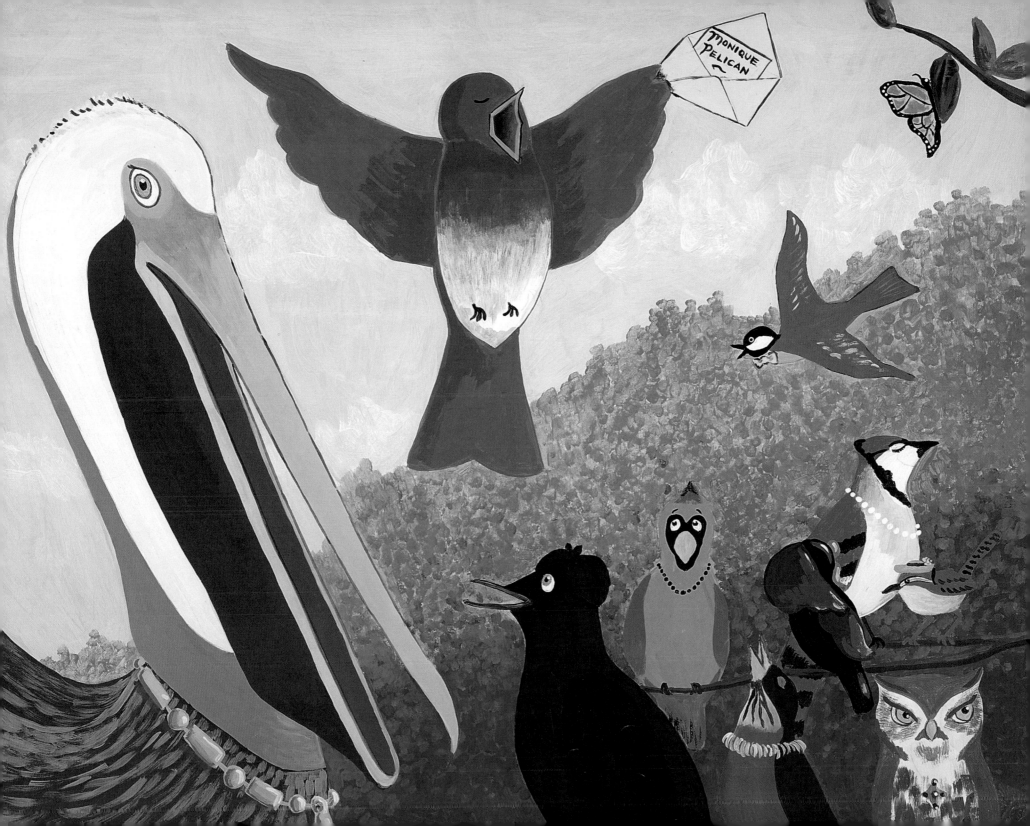

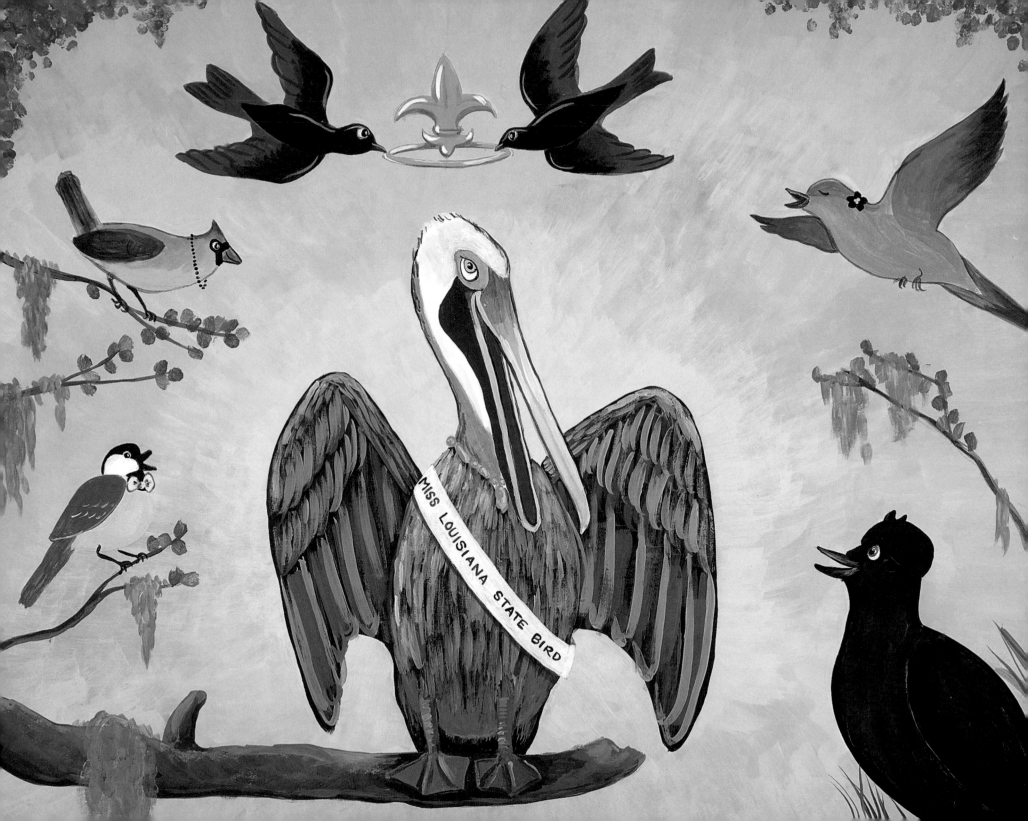

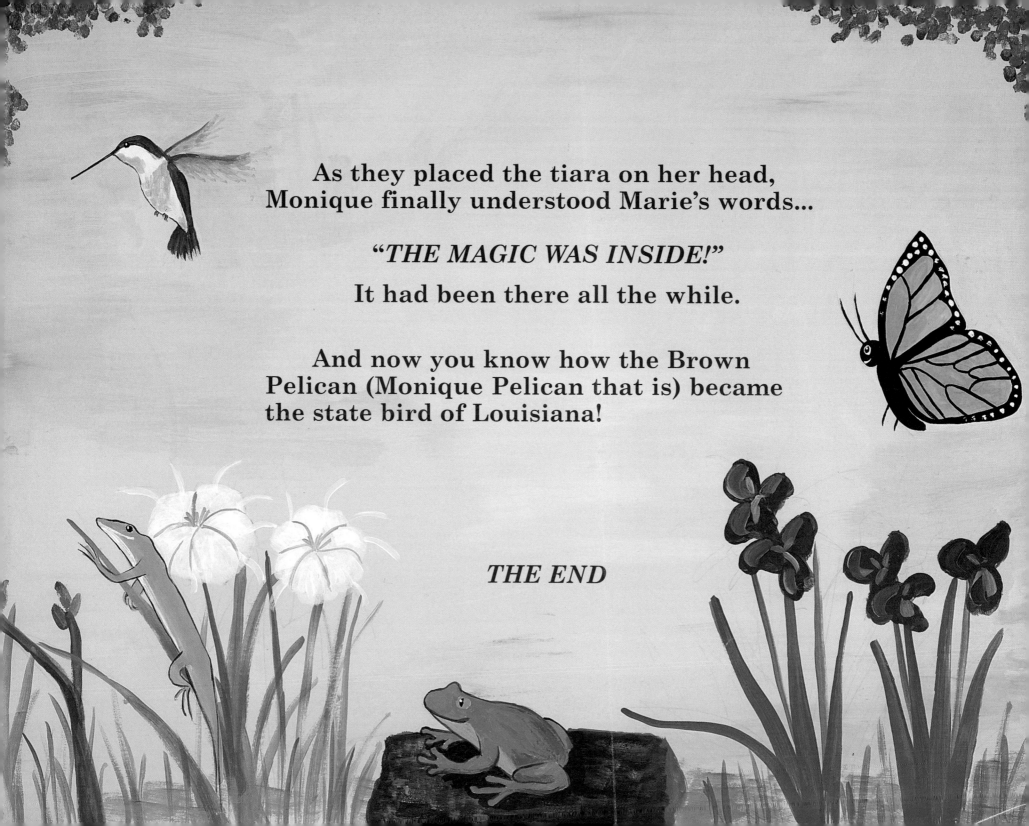

As they placed the tiara on her head, Monique finally understood Marie's words...

"THE MAGIC WAS INSIDE!"

It had been there all the while.

And now you know how the Brown Pelican (Monique Pelican that is) became the state bird of Louisiana!

THE END

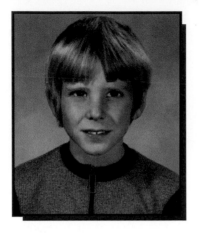

About the Author...

Todd-Michael St. Pierre is a writer and storyteller, who lives in Baton Rouge, Louisiana. He is the author of "Jambalaya, Crawfish Pie, Filé Gumbo," an internationally popular Cajun and Creole cookbook.

His Cajun heritage continues to be the inspiration for many of his stories and poems.

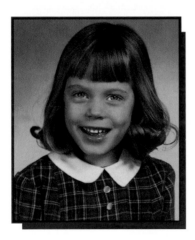

About the Illustrator...

Lori Babin Walsh always liked to draw and paint as a child, but did not become a serious artist until she grew up. This is the second book she has illustrated. She lives in Louisiana with her husband, Jeff, and children, Shannon and Sean.

SOME INTERESTING FACTS ABOUT THE BROWN PELICAN:

1. The wingspread of a Brown Pelican ranges from 6 to 7 feet, tip to tip.
2. They can fly in calm winds up to 35 miles per hour.
3. Under perfect conditions a Brown Pelican can live to be 30 plus years old.
4. A healthy adult will weigh from 6 to 10 pounds.
5. The expandable pouch below the Brown Pelican's bill can hold up to 3 times more than its stomach can.
6. Brown Pelicans plunge-dive from the air into the water for their prey—mostly fish.
7. They eat 3 to 4 pounds of fish per day.

If you would like to know more about the Brown Pelican, (Pelecanus Occidentalis) visit your local library.